WHOLE BEAUTY

Meditation & Mindfulness

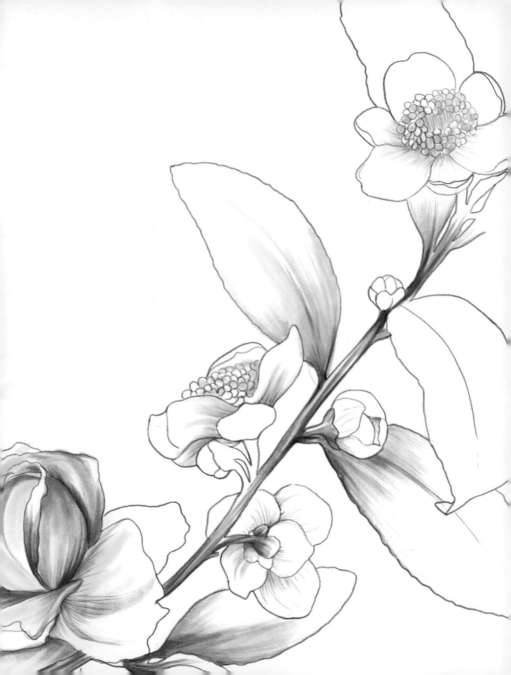

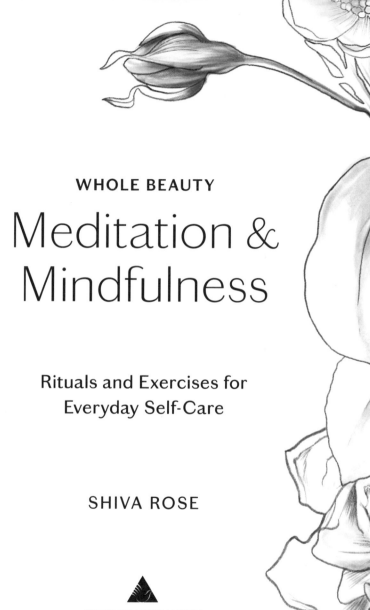

WHOLE BEAUTY

Meditation & Mindfulness

Rituals and Exercises for Everyday Self-Care

SHIVA ROSE

ARTISAN I NEW YORK

CONTENTS

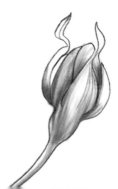

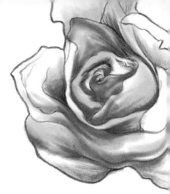

Introduction: Making Space & Time for Daily Rituals

As women, we are inherently tribal. We are meant to gather with other women, to care for one another, participate in ceremony, and be in circles. Unfortunately, we often lack this connection in our modern lives, where we work in cubicles, frequently care for our families alone, and have mothers and sisters who live far away. Our days pass without a sense of reverence and community, and we're left with a powerful yearning for connection.

Rituals provide that connection. When you perform them alone, you are able to connect with the source of all being (our own personal version of a higher power) and your deepest levels of self. When you gather for ceremony with other women, you connect with the divine feminine and form strong bonds with your teachers and friends, new sisters and mothers. Ritual and ceremony provide us with an opportunity to refuel, reenergize, and even reinvent ourselves.

When I come together with my sisters, most of the rituals we perform are very simple. We gather flowers, make a mandala, and call in the Four

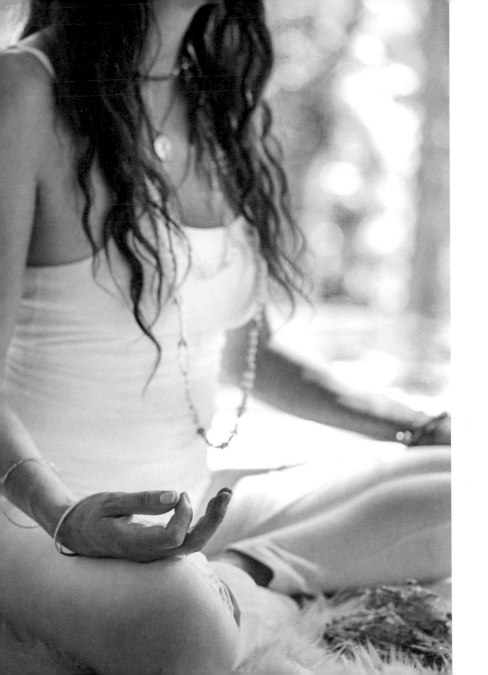

Directions, which is a Native American tradition that represents a universal way of connecting with the earth. For a small ritual, often with just one other person, a tea ceremony connects us to nature and roots us in the moment. Even just lighting a candle and saying a prayer can take ordinary life and elevate it to a higher realm. The most important thing is how you approach what you are doing.

The information in this book will guide you on your journey. But keep in mind that using your own creativity and intuition will no doubt set you on a path that is truly your own, and that's not only okay, it's also a sign that you are following your heart to the place that is right for you.

Ritual

Beautifying ourselves holistically is an integral part of self-care, health, and healing. In our modern, fast-paced era, women are stressed and under more pressure than ever before, and as a result have lost the essence of being sensual in many ways. Sensuality is about having a connection to yourself—your soul—indulging in all the things that make you feel alive and beautiful. Approaching beauty with reverence and ritual can help awaken your feminine fire and stoke the flames of vibrancy and passion. When we treat our body, our vessel, with intention, we are honoring not just ourselves but the essence of femininity that has coursed through us since the beginning of time.

Ritual is at the heart of every aspect of this book, and it is the simplest and biggest way you can honor yourself and enhance your well-being. It is the difference between rushing through a shower or bath and consciously connecting with your body; between hastily splashing on body oil and taking the time to indulge your senses and anoint yourself; between speeding through your bedtime routine and savoring it with gratitude. Mindfulness and intention are the only requirements for turning a routine into a ritual. They will transform self-care from a chore into an act of love. Creating rituals to acknowledge and induce pleasure is a form of religion, a way to care as much for the soul as for the skin. Beauty that does not penetrate beyond the first, physical layer will fade, but beauty that comes from being nourished and balanced spiritually, emotionally, and physically radiates from the eyes, hair, and every pore. Ritual helps us to create a beautiful face and a beautiful life.

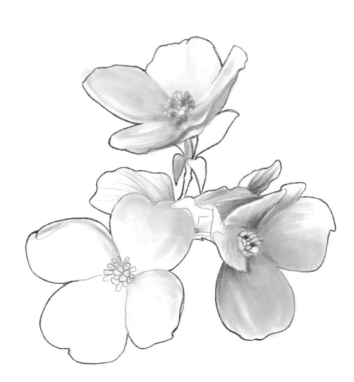

Creating a Sacred Space

The temples on either side of the forehead are reminders that we can create temples (sacred places) wherever we go just by closing our eyes and imagining them—no money or design experience needed.

However, I do think that actually creating a sacred space in your home can make you feel closer to the rituals and awaken your desire to do more. Your sacred space can be a whole room or a tiny altar on a table, but it will become the place where you apply your beauty masks, meditate, do yoga, read cards, write in your journal, or set intentions for the new moon.

An altar is the place where you'll go to connect to the source of all being and hone your intuition. As women, we're inclined to create atmosphere, we're inclined to create beauty around us, we're inclined toward being sensitive to our environment, and altars are a beautiful way to honor these inclinations.

Altars represent your life. When you clean the altar, you can imagine you're cleaning your life. When you offer flowers or fruit or incense, you're offering those to your life. Anything you do for the altar is also a meditation and intention for your life.

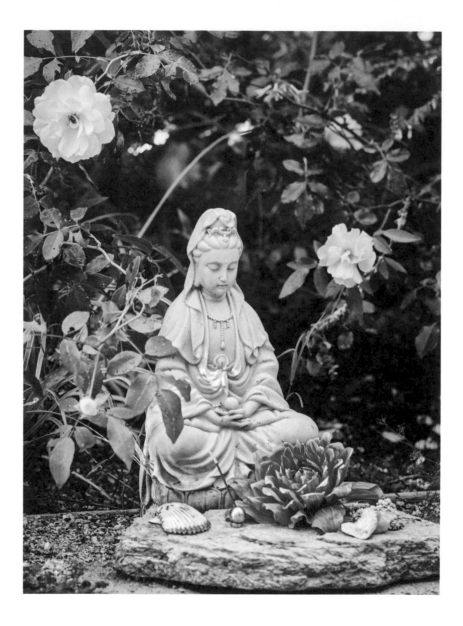

I have a few different altars. One is a nature altar, which is where I keep my crystals and things from the natural world. My children and I will add flowers in the springtime, seashells in the summer, fallen leaves in autumn, and pinecones in the winter. I have an altar to my womb, which is just a very simple space on the floor with a candle, a big rose quartz, and a beautiful piece of silk fabric. I'll light incense there, and this is where I'll sit to do my yoni egg exercises (see page 83). I have an altar for mother energy and the sacred feminine, and an altar where I practice Nichiren Buddhism. Altars should embody the idea of creating a sacred space that's just for you. An altar alters you. Virginia Woolf said that every woman needs a room of her own. I think we can adapt that sentiment and say that every woman needs an altar of her own.

Making Your Own Altar

Your altar can be as malleable and ever-changing as you are. You are not always in the same mood, dealing with the same difficulties, or pursuing the same goals, so you can adapt your altar to reflect whatever you need to honor or bring into your life at that specific point in time. There is no right or wrong way to build an altar, and the best way to do it is to let your intention guide you.

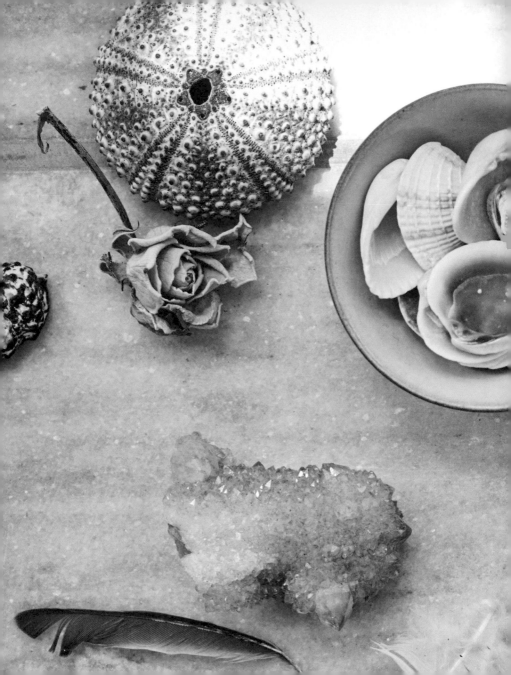

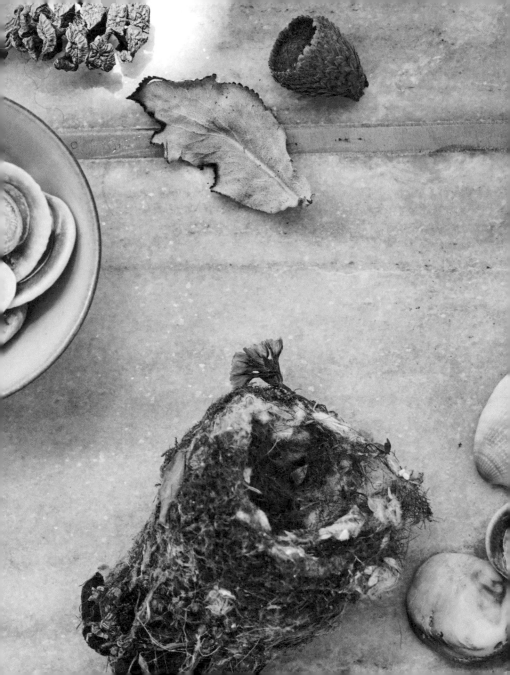

You may include any or all of the following on your altar.

- Crystals
- Flowers
- Pictures of loved ones
- Images of goddesses
- Family mementos (like a beloved relative's jewelry, or something made by your children)
- Things found in nature (rocks, feathers, shells, sticks)
- A bowl of coins (symbolizing abundance)
- Incense
- Essential oils
- A mirror (helpful for doing beauty rituals in front of the altar)
- Candles (choose the color depending on what emotion you want to bring in, a practice adopted from Wiccan literature; see opposite)

Space Clearing

The more you tune in to yourself and your own energy, the more sensitive you will become to the energy of places and other people. Whenever I come into a new space, I like to clear the energy from the past and set the stage for new blessings.

CANDLE COLORS & THEIR MEANINGS

BLACK

Removing negativity

BLUE

Peace and healing

GREEN

Prosperity

PINK

Love

PURPLE

Intuition

RED

Passion

WHITE

Blessings

YELLOW

Clarity

Thousands of years ago, people didn't believe in bacteria because they couldn't see it. I like to use that metaphor to describe energy. Just because we can't see energy doesn't mean it isn't there.

Clearing a space of previous energy is very meditative and a way of hitting reset on your mind, heart, and space. Following are a few ways to clear a space.

Sage

The burning of sage is most often associated with Native Americans, who performed ceremonial smudging to rid spaces and people of negative energy, dispel illness, and set the stage for new beginnings and good fortune. I like to accompany the act of smudging with the Native American prayer on page 20.

If you live someplace where it is easy to find wild sage, you can make your own smudge wand by binding several stems together with string and hanging it upside down to dry out. You can also dry out and burn individual leaves. Sage bundles are also easy to find at metaphysical shops, health food stores, and small gift and home shops. White sage is the type most commonly used in smudging, and you'll often find it mixed with other herbs, like sweetgrass for positive energy and juniper or cedar for healing.

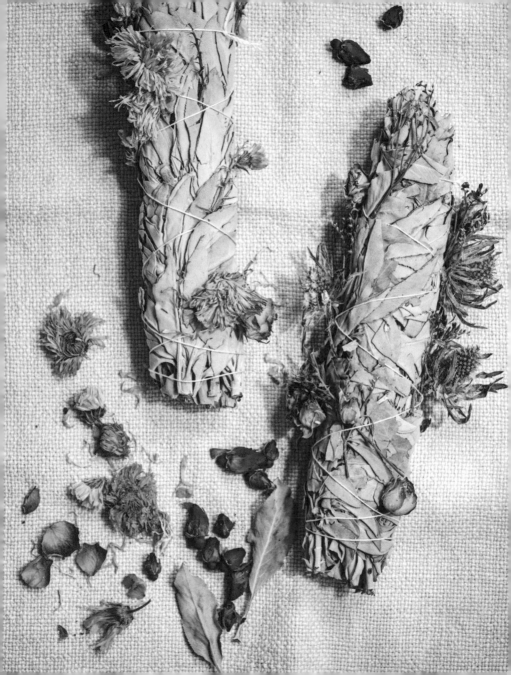

A PRAYER TO
ACCOMPANY SMUDGING

May your hands be cleansed,
that they might create beautiful things.

May your feet be cleansed,
that they might take you where you
most need to be.

May your heart be cleansed,
that you might hear its messages clearly.

May your throat be cleansed,
that you might speak rightly when
words are needed.

May your eyes be cleansed,
that you might see the signs and
wonders of the world.

May this person and space be washed clean
by the smoke of these fragrant plants.

And may that same smoke carry your prayers,
spiraling, to the heavens.

Burn your sage in a heatproof container to catch all the ash and embers. An abalone shell is traditional, but you can also use a copper bowl, a terra-cotta pot, or any other vessel that is safe and also pleasing to you.

Light the sage, and when it goes out (you may have to blow on it) and starts to smoke, use your hand, a feather, or another lightweight object to disperse the smoke into all four corners of the room and around your altar while imagining all of the energy of the past being carried away with the drifting smoke. Make sure all the doors and windows are open.

You can also burn sage when recovering from an illness, after an argument with your significant other, or any time you feel the need to refresh and reset your environment. You can smudge people too, by sweeping the smoke along their limbs, across their body, and under their feet.

Salt

Salt is able to absorb and trap negative energy that is released from people, objects, and events.

The easiest way to clear a space with salt is to place small bowls in each corner of the room, mindfully stating your intention as you do so. I like to say, "I

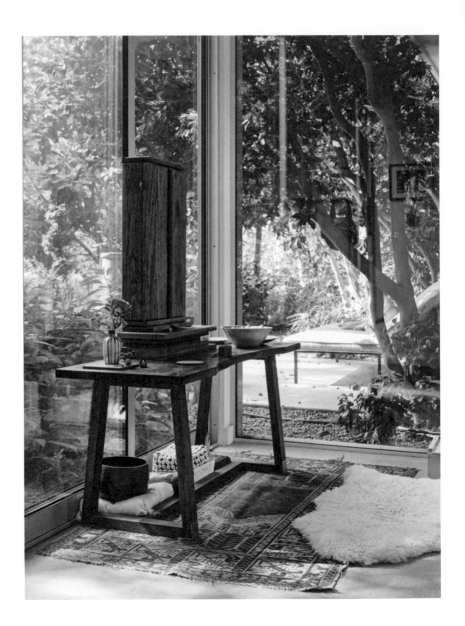

cleanse this room of any impurities, negativity, or anything that doesn't support my highest good. Amen." Leave the salt for twenty-four hours, then bury it or throw it into the ocean. You can do this whenever you move into a new home, before rituals, or after stressful situations in the home.

Incense

The burning of incense as part of ceremony and ritual is something that you will find across cultures and religions. In Buddhist temples, circular coils of incense are burned to bring forth bodhisattvas and other deities. In Christian and Jewish ceremonies, incense is lit so that the burning smoke may represent the prayers of the faithful rising to heaven. In Hinduism, incense is often a daily offering to a god, and on a Wiccan altar, a lit stick of incense represents the element of air.

Incense was often crafted from whatever materials were available locally, like wood, bark, flowers, resin, or roots, so the types of incense used during rituals differed greatly from region to region.

Use any type of nontoxic incense that is pleasing to you in form and scent. After cleansing, the burning of incense welcomes in angels, ancestors, and spirits to bring blessings and guide you on your way.

Cedar or Pine

These woodsy scents smell clean and fresh,
and they clear negative energy.

Copal

Smoky and lush, copal powerfully
cleanses spaces and auras.

Frankincense

This sweet scent is used for purification
and heightened spirituality. It traditionally
represents masculine energy.

Myrrh

An earthy, almost anise scent that is used to
bring in positive energy, myrrh traditionally
is seen as a representation of feminine
energy. Frankincense and myrrh are often
burned or blended together to balance
masculine and feminine energy.

New Mexico Piñon

This incense is made from an evergreen tree
that grows in New Mexico, Arizona, Texas,
and Wyoming. When burned, it has a beautiful
woodsy scent. It was traditionally lit during
Native American ceremonies for protection.
Prayers can be sent through the smoke.

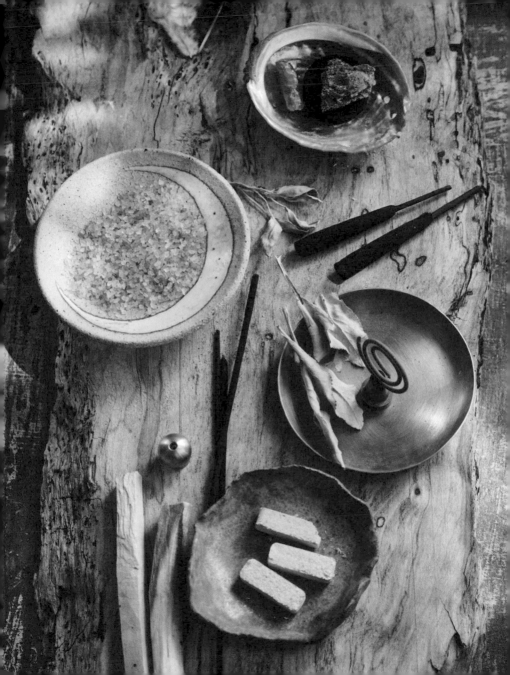

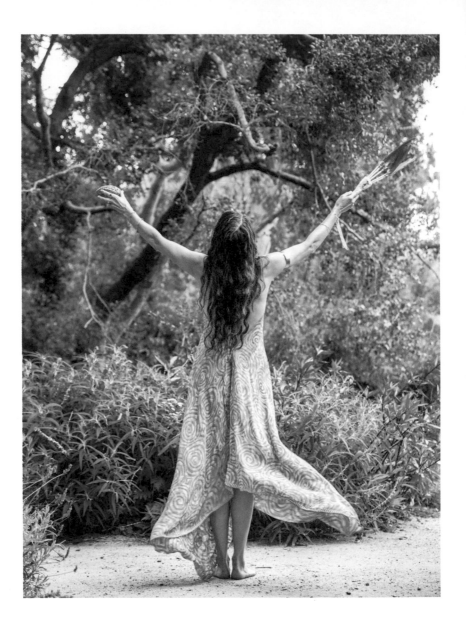

Calling In the Four Directions

For bigger rituals, like a circle with friends, celebrating the new or full moon with my sisters, or the beginning of a retreat, I will call in the Four Directions. This is a Native American prayer that honors the elements and pays homage to the belief that all life is interconnected. We humans are an integral part of nature, so every time we honor Mother Earth, we are also honoring ourselves. Begin by facing east, then turn your body ninety degrees with each new verse, completely opening the space so that the divine force may enter it to bless you.

A Prayer to Call In the Four Directions

Great spirits of the east, the land of the rising sun, the land of new beginnings. The land of the great condor and the eagle, please join me here today in this sacred space. Please bring me your energy, please protect me under your wings as the great condor does. Please let me see the great perspective of my life from the heights of the eagle and the condor. Thank you for being here today, great spirits of the east.

Great spirits of the south, the land of fire, the land of ambition, the land of desire, sexuality, fertility. Thank you for being here today with me.

The land of the great serpent, please allow me to shed what no longer serves me, as a snake does. Please allow the coils of the light and the coils of protection to surround me here today. Great spirits of the south, please ignite my passion and my ambition for the betterment of this planet. Thank you, great spirits of the south.

Great spirits of the west, the land of the setting sun, the land of dreams, the land of the unconscious, the land of water. Thank you for being here today with me. I want to give a blessing of gratitude for all the rains you have brought us. I would like to honor all the ways in which water blesses my life. The land of the jaguar, the land of medicine, please be here with me today. Thank you, great spirits of the west.

Great spirits of the north, the land of the ancestors. Thank you for all my ancestors, seven generations past. Thank you for protecting me, and for the seven generations to come. Thank you for being here today, hummingbird medicine, bear medicine, all that come from the north. Let me be able to take in the sweet nectar of my life, as the hummingbird takes in nectar from the flowers. Let me have the strength and wisdom of the bear. Thank you, great winds and spirits of the north.

Great Mama Earth, Pachamama, Gaia, thank you for being here today with me. Thank you for all your blessings, thank you for the mountains, the rivers, the streams, the creeks. Thank you for all your creatures, the two-legged, the four-legged, the creepy-crawlies, the winged ones, the finned ones. Thank you. Thank you for protecting us. I offer to be a guardian for you. I offer to bring you protection. Thank you for being here today with me, O great spirit of Mother Earth.

Great spirits of the sky, Father Sky, Mother Moon, Sister Wind, Star Nation People, thank you for all your energy, celestial beings. Thank you for shining your light among us. Thank you for being here today with me.

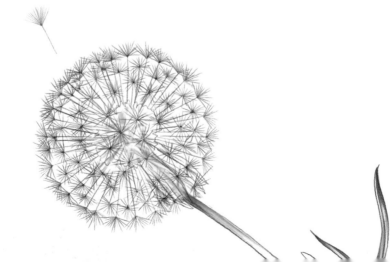

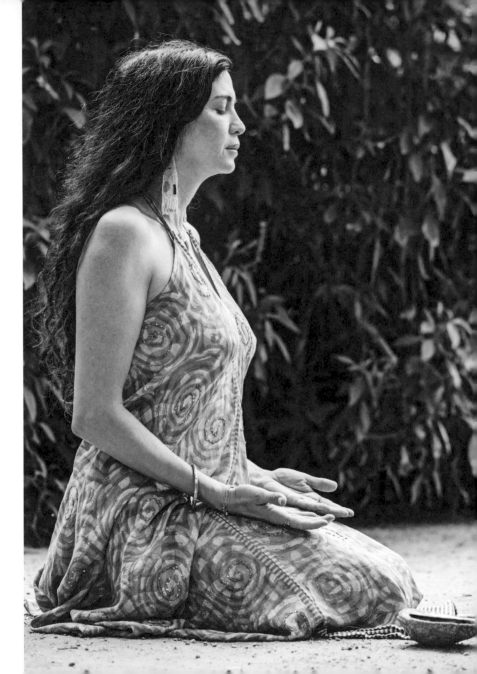

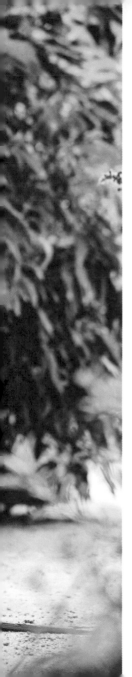

At the end of the ritual, it is important to close the space, so you can conclude with something very simple:

Thank you for being with us today, great spirits of the east, great spirits of the south, great spirits of the west, great spirits of the north, and the celestial mothers and fathers. Thank you.

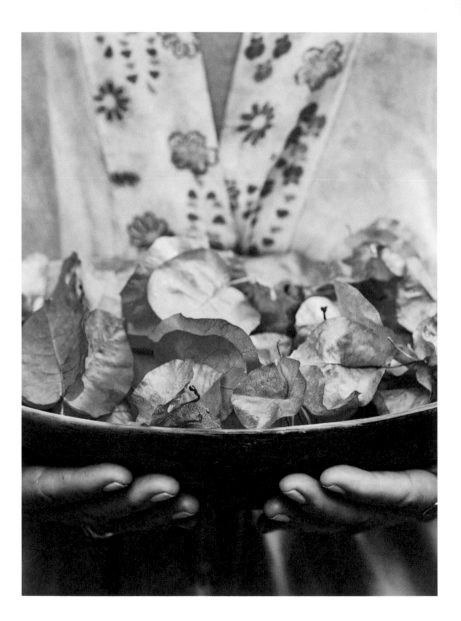

A Simple Ritual Opening

Sometimes you don't have the time or space for
a full ritual but still want to honor something
with an intention. In those moments, you can
use these simple words to bring mindfulness
and awareness to any ritual or practice.

*I am now connecting to the source, the source of
all being, and I'm asking that my heart be open for
this ritual that I'm about to begin. I want to thank
all my guides that watch over me and all the earth's
energy that watches over me. I want to be able to fill
myself with love and abundance and the light of the
universe. I am bountiful, I am blissful, I am beautiful.*

Honoring Nature with Ritual

Women have their own cycles and are very connected to the cycles of nature as well. When we go on walks, my daughters and I will bring home things to put on our altar. In the fall, these may be acorns or pinecones; in the springtime, blossoms or seeds. We'll add driftwood, seashells, and rocks—one of my most precious possessions is my collection of heart-shaped rocks! We also like to honor the changing seasons with rituals that remind us to care for the earth as we care for ourselves.

Spring

Spring is all about rebirth, regrowth, and renewal. This is the time of year when the world explodes with the scent and color of flowers. When you are hiking, or at home in your garden, you can imprint this beauty on your soul by laying out a mandala of petals, sticks, leaves, rocks, and whatever else may be easily accessible. It is a very meditative practice. The mandala can be shaped like a star, heart, flower, or design of your choosing. Let your creativity flow, and you will soon find that you are concentrating not on the trivial to-dos of the day but on the textures of nature.

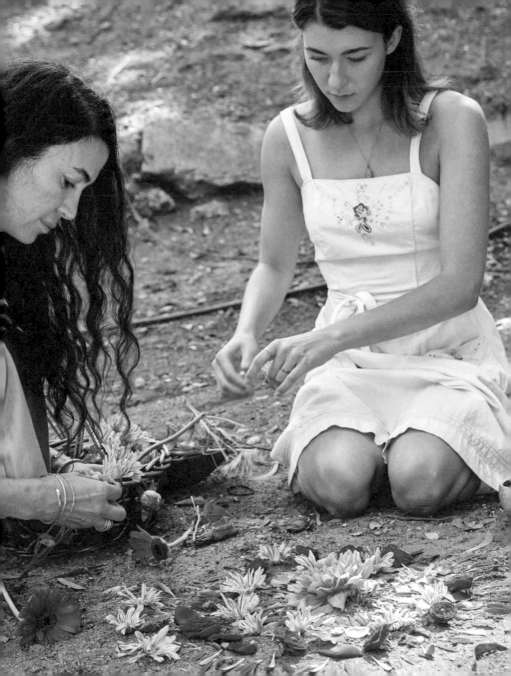

Summer

Summer is a time to express gratitude and pay homage to all that you have harvested. Feast on cool, juicy fruits. Whenever you can, sit by still water to meditate (even a pool will do). Since your skin is likely to be dehydrated from the sun and the heat, do what you can to replenish moisture. Break out your hydrosols (water infused with flowers, herbs, or essential oils) and mist yourself throughout the day, expressing reverence for the water each time you do.

Autumn

Autumn is a time for hearth and home and making preparations for winter. It's about getting ready to rest and hibernate. Look forward to gathering wood for cozy fires, and planting bulbs that will bloom in the spring. With the holidays on the horizon, autumn is a time for gatherings. Sage your space (see page 18) and host circles, inviting people into your home to share energy and create warmth. Autumn is also the ideal time to journal, both to reflect on the year that has passed and to anticipate the one to come. A great way to begin the journaling practice is by setting aside a few minutes first thing in the morning or before you go to bed at night to write whatever comes into

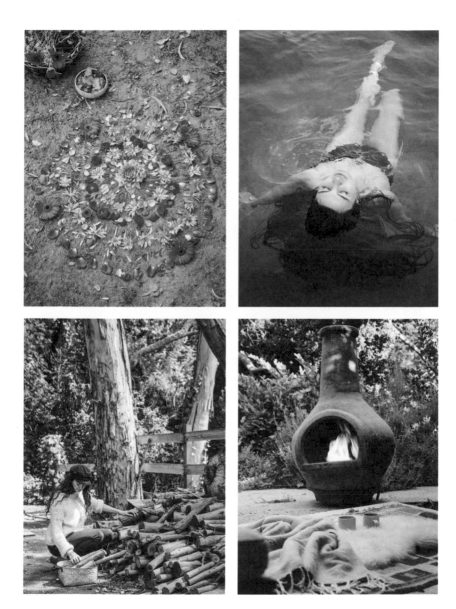

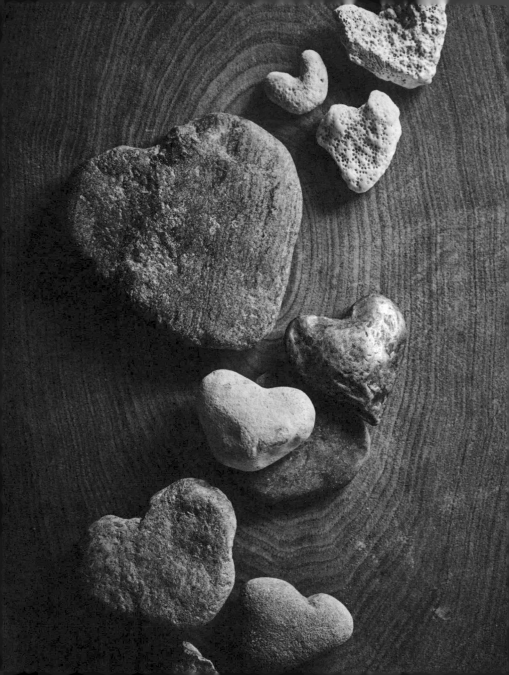

your head. Start with as little as five minutes, and don't judge or edit the words as they flow from your hand onto the page. Just write. Increase the time if you have a desire to continue writing.

Winter

Winter is a time to nourish yourself and regain your strength. There is something so beautiful about living in sync with nature, and in winter you can be as quiet as the snow-covered ground. Hibernate. Eat root vegetables to ground yourself to the earth, make soups to nourish yourself and those you care about, and light candles to bring warmth into your home. If you are the type to bundle up and go for walks outdoors, you can look for treasures and make winter mandalas with pinecones, evergreen branches, and winter berries.

Phases of the Moon

Birth, life, death, and renewal are all reflected
in the cycle of the moon, and menstrual
cycles often mirror the moon's cycle.

The new moon is a time for starting projects and
increasing abundance. It is also a good time to do an
intention-setting ritual, writing down your intentions
on a piece of paper, then waiting until a full moon
to throw the paper into a fire to release them.
The full moon is a time for healing rituals, finishing
projects, and gathering the moon's energy. The
waning moon is a time for clearing and cleansing.

Timing your beauty rituals to coincide with the
phases of different moons can be a powerful way
to reconnect with nature and the cycles within
your life. I like to use scrubs on the new moon, then
replenish with nourishing masks on the full moon.

Native Americans had different names for each full
moon, and the names often varied depending on tribe
and region. Consider adding a moon calendar to your
sacred space (there are several beautiful, artisan-
designed ones available), and let these names guide
what you add to your altar throughout the year.

JANUARY
Wolf Moon

FEBRUARY
Snow Moon

MARCH
Worm Moon

APRIL
Pink Moon

MAY
Flower Moon

JUNE
Strawberry Moon

JULY
Thunder Moon

AUGUST
Sturgeon Moon

SEPTEMBER
Corn Moon

OCTOBER
Hunter's Moon

NOVEMBER
Frost Moon

DECEMBER
Long Nights Moon

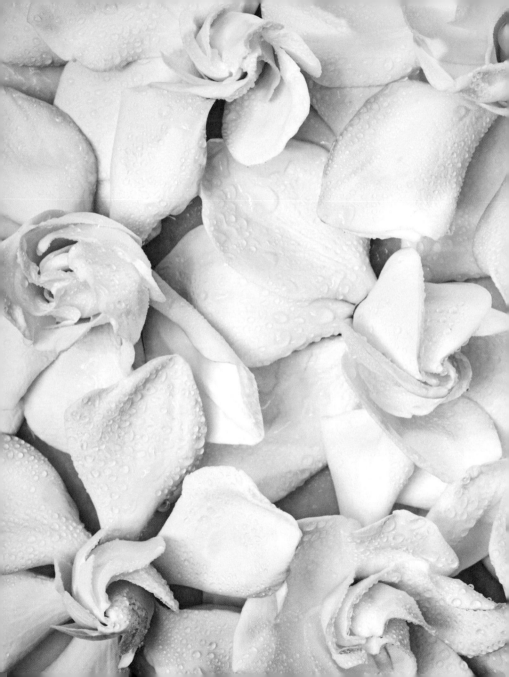

Ayurvedic Practices

Inner and outer beauty are intimately related. Ayurveda, a science of self-healing, encompasses diet, meditation, breathing techniques, medicinal herbs, beauty practices, and rituals to heal the body, mind, and spirit.

Ayurvedic medicine has a rich history, which was originally passed on through the oral tradition, then later recorded in Sanskrit in the four sacred texts called the Vedas. This ancient practice is all about connecting to ourselves and staying balanced and in harmony with the natural world. In sharp contrast to Western medicine, Ayurveda is preventive, with the focus on constantly cleansing and detoxifying the body through practices like oil pulling (see page 48) and dry brushing (see page 49) and by following a holistic diet. But Ayurvedic practices aren't just about preventing diseases rather than simply curing them; they're also about how to live in a state of vigor and energy. In India, more than 90 percent of the population uses some form of Ayurvedic medicine. While it's becoming much more popular here in the West, it's still considered an alternative approach.

The theory behind Ayurveda is that all areas of life impact one's health. Here in the Western world, we believe in using targeted tactics—generally, prescription medications—to cure specific ailments. Ayurveda views the body as a whole. Like traditional Chinese medicine, it is about the mind, body, and spirit connection.

The aim of Ayurveda is to return the body to its original healthy state; true luminous beauty must be supported by health. At the heart of Ayurveda are *ojas*, our life force, the very essence of our health and well-being. They are our honey, the sap in the tree that is our body. Ojas give us the ability to thrive. When our ojas are strong, our bodies are firm and flexible, our skin is clear and glowing, and our hair is shiny and healthy. Ojas also allow us to overflow with love and compassion.

However, the modern world takes its toll on ojas. Constant stress, processed food, technology, overextension, and too much information deplete ojas and dry them out. When we restore them—with meditation, healthy food, and being in tune with the universe—we become radiant.

Ridding your body of waste and toxins helps ojas to flourish, as detoxing allows the system to be nourished. When your body is clear of toxins, it is able to receive the healthy benefits of nutritious food, face masks, and body oils. Rather than promote a harsh, all-at-once approach to detoxing, Ayurveda employs several small daily or weekly practices to help ensure that your body is always being cleansed and efficiently processing waste.

Slowly incorporate these practices into your day. You can begin with something as small as integrating fresh produce into your diet, massaging your feet before bed, or dry brushing your skin in the morning. These additions to your routine will help you to continuously keep your body in a rhythm and in balance. Once you know your body, you can adjust certain practices. Following are some that I try to incorporate into my day. I alter them depending on how much time I have and if I am traveling.

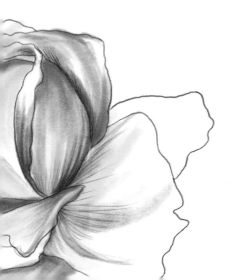

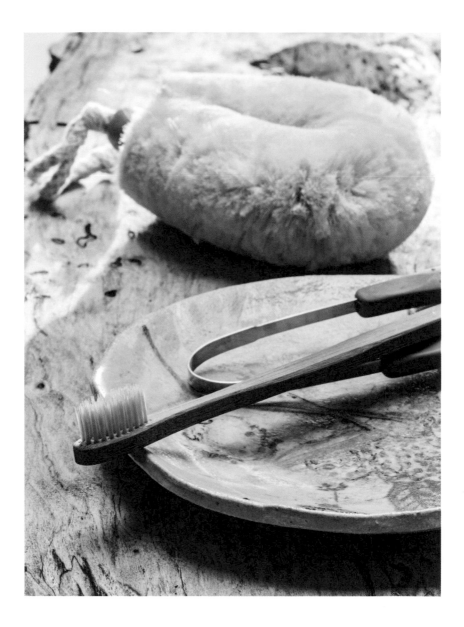

Tongue Scraping

Scraping your tongue every morning can give you clues as to how efficiently your digestive system is functioning. If your tongue is very coated, it usually means there is a lot of *ama*, or toxicity, in your system.

TO PRACTICE TONGUE SCRAPING:

- Use a stainless-steel tongue scraper (which you can find online or in most health food stores) or a spoon. Gently scrape from the back or base of the tongue forward until you have scraped the whole surface, which is typically accomplished with anywhere between seven and fourteen strokes. This clears away any bacteria. Scraping stimulates the gastric and digestive enzymes to wake up and start working.

- Rinse out your mouth, and proceed with oil pulling.

Oil Pulling

During the night, as you sleep, your body builds up toxins while it is in the resting, cleansing state. Oil pulling allows these toxins to be released. It should be done first thing in the morning, before you have anything to drink or eat, and ideally after scraping your tongue. Coconut, sunflower, and sesame oil all work well, but coconut oil has the added benefit of whitening your teeth.

TO PRACTICE OIL PULLING:

- Take a spoonful of oil and swish it in your mouth for fifteen to twenty minutes. (This is the recommended period of time, but you can also do it for just a few minutes to feel and see the freshening and teeth-whitening effects of the coconut oil.)

- It is important to keep the oil in your mouth and not swallow it. It also is wise to spit it out in either the toilet or a trash can, as it can clog a sink.

- After you finish pulling, brush your teeth or rinse out your mouth very well.

Dry Brushing

The skin is our largest organ and is responsible for 25 percent of the body's ability to detox, yet we tend to focus our beauty routines on the face and hands when the whole body deserves reverence and respect. In addition to being an Ayurvedic practice, skin brushing for the whole body has been used for ages in Scandinavia, Russia, Japan, and Greece and by the Cherokee tribe (using dried corncobs), to name just a few examples. Dry brushing helps rid the body of dead skin and also stimulates the lymphatic and circulatory systems, which assist the kidneys and liver in releasing excess hormones that have built up in the organs.

Over time, dry brushing can prevent cellulite and help regenerate collagen, and in the short term, it invigorates and energizes you. As you are shedding dead skin, you are also releasing that which no longer serves you. Dry brushing should be done before bathing or showering.

Continued

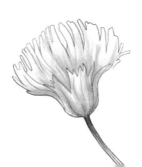

TO PRACTICE DRY BRUSHING:

- Using a body brush with natural bristles (I like ones that have copper in them to help balance electromagnetic fields), start at the feet and move up toward the torso.

- Using long strokes in the direction of your heart, brush each part of the body six times.

- Brush so it feels slightly painful but good—like when you do a really deep stretch.

- To increase the detoxifying effects, follow with a cold shower.

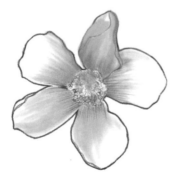

Self-Massage

In the West, we consider a massage to be a special treat, but for many in India, massages are a regular part of life. Babies and toddlers are massaged daily, and when they are a little bit older, they are taught to massage their family members. Women get daily massages for forty days after giving birth. Once you become accustomed to the health and beauty benefits of massages, you won't be able to do without them. Fortunately for our wallets, Ayurveda considers self-massage, or *abhyanga*, to be just as beneficial as a massage given by another.

Set aside some time once a week, or daily if you can, to practice abhyanga, and you will soon see the benefits, including toned, glowing skin; improved circulation; the relief of stiffness in the joints; and the flushing out of toxins in the body. It's also a wonderful way to get to know your own body better.

Use sesame, sunflower, or almond oil for massage. It feels extra luxurious if you warm it beforehand. Put the oil in a glass bowl. Heat a few inches of water in a saucepan and place the bowl in the water for a few minutes, until the oil is warm.

Continued

- Apply warm oil generously to your body, beginning with your limbs. Use long strokes on your arms and legs and circular motions on your joints. Massage clockwise to release tension, and include areas like your neck and under your arms to target lymph nodes.

- Massage your abdomen and chest in broad clockwise, circular motions. Follow the path of the intestine on your stomach, moving up on the right side, then down on the left.

- Apply oil to your crown chakra, at the top of your head, working outward in circular motions.

- Dip your fingertips in the oil and massage your ears.

- Massage your feet (but make sure to wipe off the oil before you walk).

- Throughout the massage, send loving intentions to your organs and show gratitude to your body for everything it does for you.

- Allow enough time for the oil to soak into your skin before you dress.

If you don't have time for a full massage, you can always take a small scoop of shea butter and give yourself a foot massage before bed. This serves as a form of acupressure, and the shea butter helps moisturize dry skin. At the same time, you're honoring your feet—which are your foundation—and how much they do for you throughout the day.

A note on chakras: Chakra *means "wheel" in Sanskrit, and the chakras are the seven turning wheels of our energy field (or subtle body). The chakras can be found from the top of the head down to the bottom of the spine. When they are active and spinning, they brighten our aura. When they are closed and stagnant, our aura dims. When our chakras are balanced and working together, we feel confident, calm, and energized, both grounded and in touch with our divine self.*

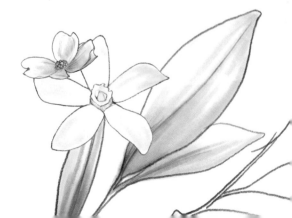

Facial Steaming

Facial steaming is wonderful to do before a bath or shower. It opens your pores, which helps to get rid of impurities and enables your facial products to be absorbed more easily; afterward, you'll be glowing. Steaming also can be a meditative time when you visualize all the incredible properties of the plants nourishing your skin and soul. Make your own custom facial steam by mixing wonderfully fragrant dried herbs with beautiful, colorful flowers. Look for ones that are organic and pesticide-free from a trusted source.

If you can't grow your own herbs and flowers or get them from someone you know, I recommend trying Mountain Rose Herbs (see Resources).

TO PRACTICE FACIAL STEAMING:

- Thoroughly cleanse your face.

- Boil three cups of water in a pot. Remove the pot from the heat and pour the water into a bowl.

- Add three tablespoons of a mix of herbs and flowers, and three to five drops of essential oil (if using). A little goes a long way.

Continued

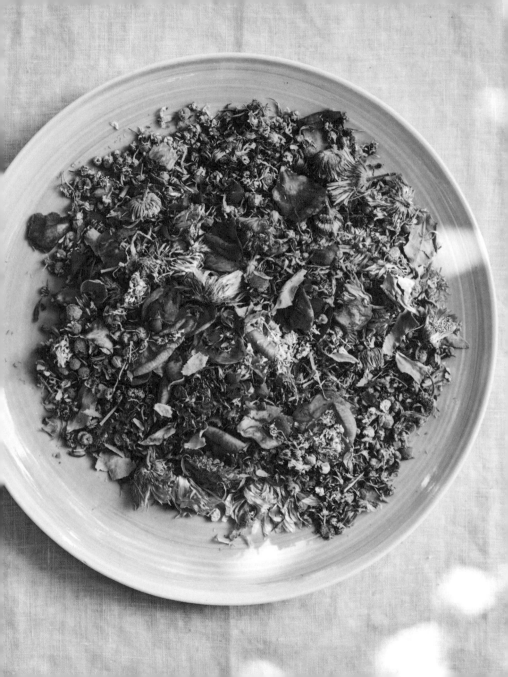

- Cover and let steep for five minutes.

- Place your face over the bowl, and using a towel or cloth, create a tent to trap the steam.

- Sit for ten minutes, relaxing and visualizing beautiful images. (I like to think of being bathed in nourishing rays of light, almost as if I am under a waterfall.)

- Rinse your face with cool water.

- Follow with moisturizer or face oil.

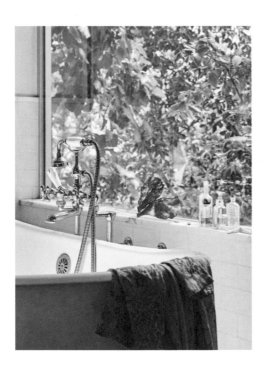

Calendula

Moisturizes dry skin and has anti-aging properties

Chamomile

Acts as an anti-inflammatory and prevents wrinkles

Cornflower

Soothes and decongests the skin, acts as an
astringent, and lightens the complexion

Dandelion

Releases impurities

Raspberry Leaf

Soothes sensitive skin and balances hormones

Rose Petals

Act as an anti-inflammatory and
help with sun damage

Sage

Improves circulation

Yarrow

Heals wounds and enhances circulation

ESSENTIAL OILS
FOR STEAMING

Bergamot • Neroli • Rose • Sandalwood

Honoring Our Connection to the Natural World

Ayurveda flourished at a time when humans were more connected to the natural world around them. The rhythms of the day were more related to the seasons and the cycles of human life. Modern advances have caused us to lose our essential connection with the earth, but when we make a point of seeking to regain that connection, our rhythms become more fluid and in tune with natural cycles. We can do this by spending time outdoors. If we live in a city, we can visit nearby parks and be among trees, plants, and flowers. If we live by canyons or an ocean, then we can make time each day to connect there with the source of all being. Listen to the sounds and smell the scents of nature, and honor yourself by honoring the cycles and bounty of Mother Earth.

Earthing

One way to connect with nature is simply to walk barefoot. We used to be in almost constant contact with the earth through the soles of our feet, but now we spend most of our time indoors or in shoes. Earthing is an Ayurvedic practice that

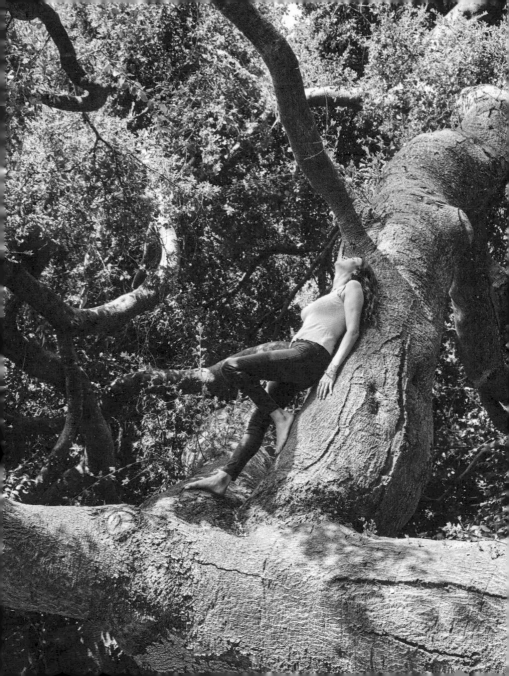

many use to connect with nature. Simply going barefoot outside can help you reestablish that bond. Our feet are actually portals to health, and through them, we can take in the natural minerals and enzymes of the earth. Doing so helps lower heart rate, decrease inflammation, calm the nervous system, and stimulate pressure points that can improve circulation. The Japanese have a special term for the healing and cleansing power of nature: *shinrin-yoku*, which means "forest-bathing." Even if you can't go barefoot, taking a walk in the woods will do wonders for your whole being.

Kundalini &
Mindfulness
Practices

Kundalini is a physical and spiritual practice. It combines yoga poses with meditations in the form of *kriya*. *Kriya* means "action," and it uses a series of postures, breath, and sound to trigger a physiological reaction in the brain that helps to change negative thought patterns to positive ones. Mantras can have the same effect through the use of sound. Kundalini employs mantras to "tune in" to the divine that is within all of us.

According to Yogi Bhajan, who is credited with bringing Kundalini to the United States, it is a "technology" that you can use to set change in motion. It replaces your old conditioning and generates self-love. Kundalini mantras, such as "I am bountiful, I am blissful, I am beautiful," resonate with people from all walks of life in their beauty and simplicity, and if you say those words often enough, you will start to believe them! I truly believe that there is no outer beauty without inner beauty, and inner beauty starts with a compassionate heart and a mind that is free from fear, worry, and stress—plus we all know stress accelerates aging!

Kundalini derives its name through its focus on awakening the spiritual energy that is coiled like a snake (a literal translation of the Sanskrit term *kundalini*) at the base of the spine, through regularly practicing meditation, *pranayama* (breathing techniques), yoga asanas, and chanting mantras. Referred to as "the yoga of awareness" by practitioners, it aims—according to one of my teachers—"to cultivate the creative spiritual potential of a human to uphold values, speak truth, and focus on the compassion and consciousness needed to serve and heal others." When you are engaged in Kundalini, you have to be present—your brain doesn't really have a choice. The reason Kundalini is so effective is because it's physiological. It works on the adrenals, it works on the hormones, it works on the pituitary—it actually works on the entire glandular system. There are a lot of variations of yoga out there, but I feel that when people come into Kundalini, they really notice a difference, a shift in their life and mind-set.

It is a long-held belief that it takes forty days to change a pattern of behavior. With the first twenty, you're breaking old habits. With the second, you're forming new ones. I always tell people who aren't sure about meditation to try it for forty days and see what happens. The time will pass before you know it, there's no risk of harm, and chances are you will notice profound differences in your life.

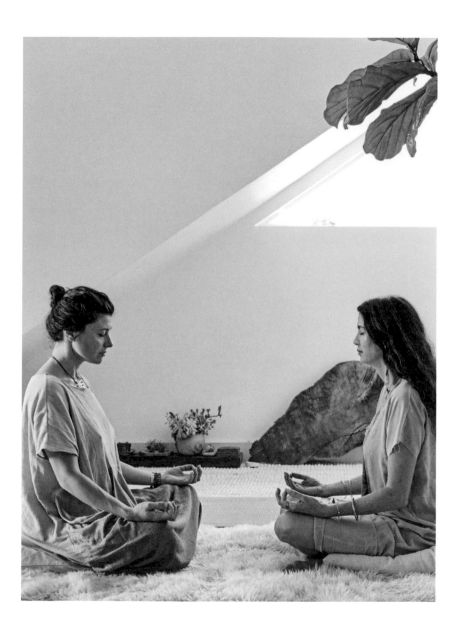

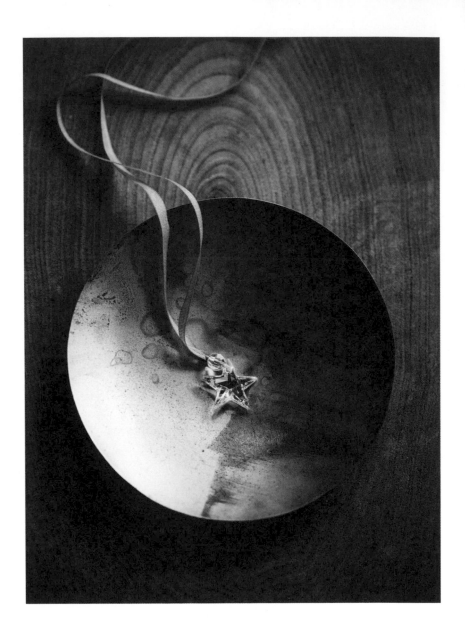

Guided Meditations

These visualizations and meditations are an easy
introduction to the practice, and the more you
do them, the calmer your mind will become and
the easier meditating will be. Many people are
intimidated by meditation because they think it
involves sitting still and in silence for twenty minutes
or more. While you will work up to that with some
meditations, you can start with these active ones
and do them for just a few minutes or rounds of
breath. It really is up to you. Some people may
find one minute challenging; others may be able
to sit for much longer without feeling anxious.

Find a comfortable place to sit or lie, and set a timer.
For the duration of that time frame, try to be mindful
and focus on the meditation. If your mind drifts, don't
berate yourself. Just gently return your focus to the
meditation and continue. You do not have to do the
same meditation every day, though you certainly can,
and you can also do different ones in succession.

Guiding Star Meditation

This is great to do when you are dealing with
challenges or negative situations and need to

be reminded of your powerful inner light and to increase self-love and positivity. As women, we hold a lot of our power in our belly, in our sacrum. Begin by imagining a star there, to increase your positive power, or in your heart, to increase love.

Picture a tiny crystal that is no more than a pinpoint of light. Close your eyes and breathe in and out through your nose.

With each breath, imagine the pinpoint of light growing and getting bigger, until it is a big star right in the middle of your belly or your chest. Imagine all of the rays of the star extending out from you, sharing your beautiful golden light with the world. With every breath, focus on the star. See how it is shiny, bright, sparkly, and white with positivity. It is radiating love.

Imagine each of the star's rays sending that love to the people you care about. I see the rays encompassing my children, my animals, and my home, then my extended family, my work, my friends, and my business. The rays keep growing, until I send my light to my city, our country, the world, and the entire planet.

The star has now become a bright golden light that encompasses everything, sending healing love to all corners of the earth. From there, I start to bring it back in. The star gets smaller and smaller with each breath, until it is the size of a silver dollar. Then I

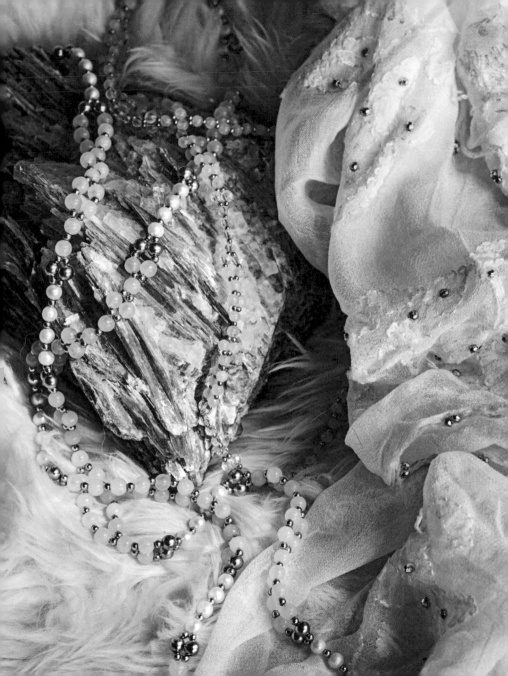

let it rest right there, in my chest or my belly, as my power center that lets me carry that healing light and love with me for the rest of my day.

Empowering White Light Meditation

This Kundalini-based meditation is a good one to do first thing in the morning to set the course of your day. It floods your body with healing energy, leaving no space for negativity, and illuminates the shadows—think of it as turning on a light to show your children that there is nothing fearsome hiding in the closet. Just as the sun gives the earth the light that allows things to grow, this meditation similarly nourishes mind and body.

Sit comfortably with your arms upstretched in a "V." Close your eyes and breathe normally. Begin by imagining a beam of light coming into your body through your crown chakra at the top of your head. Imagine the light traveling down to your third eye, located in the center of your forehead, and blessing all of your dreams and visions. (The third eye, which is right where your pituitary gland is, is associated with the god Shiva and has been called the "gateway to the unconscious" because it is the seat of our intuition.)

From there, it progresses into your throat, onto your shoulders, and down your arms. Imagine the white

light bathing you all the way to the tips of
your fingers.

Allow the light to enter and heal your heart,
then travel down through your stomach to
your root chakra (located in the sacral area
around the groin), making you feel grounded
and supported. Allow it to travel through your
legs, down to your feet and into your toes.

While you are doing this, repeat "Receive,
receive, receive" as the light fills you up.

When you feel that the light has illuminated every
part of your body, hold it there for a second,
being grateful for how blessed and protected
you are in everything you do. Then bring your
hands down, outstretched, on either side of your
body. As you do so, imagine you're cleansing your
aura, sweeping it clean of debris and baggage,
negative energy, mental anguish—whatever
you're carrying that no longer serves you. Then
put your hands on the ground and imagine that
you're releasing whatever you don't want anymore
into the earth, which is taking it in for you.

This little meditation fills your body with
energy and snaps you out of depression or
sadness. It is hard to be down after doing it.

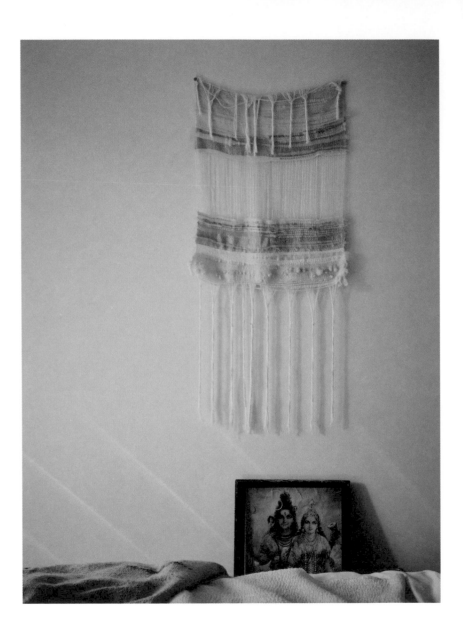

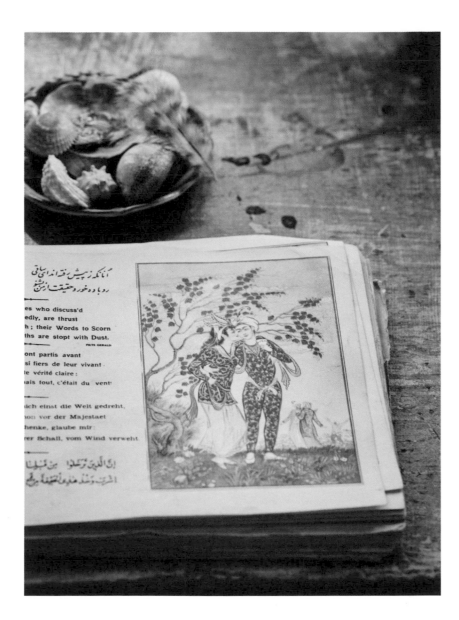

es who discuss'd
edly, are thrust
h; their Words to Scorn
ths are stopt with Dust.
                    FITZ GERALD

ont partis avant
si fiers de leur vivant:
le vérité claire:
ais tout, c'était du vent'

ich einst die Welt gedreht,
oo vor der Majestaet
henke, glaube mir:
rer Schall, vom Wind verweht

Breathing

Prana, or "breath," is what fuels our life force. Most of us aren't taught how to breathe correctly and usually only do so in a shallow manner. Once you learn to fill your diaphragm and lungs with air, you will notice how much more awake you feel. These yogic breathing methods are also anti-aging because they help awaken the endocrine system and bring more oxygen to the skin and organs.

Breath of Fire

In Kundalini yoga, it is said that if you feel down or depressed, it's because you don't have enough prana in your system. Breath of fire, a Kundalini kriya (exercise), remedies this. It is a vehicle for changing your brain chemistry and creating lots of joyful energy.

For breath of fire, sit in a comfortable position holding your arms up in a "V." Close the four fingers of each hand against your palms, and have your thumbs out, pointing in toward each other.

Inhale and exhale through your nose, rapidly, and with enough force that you feel your diaphragm moving.

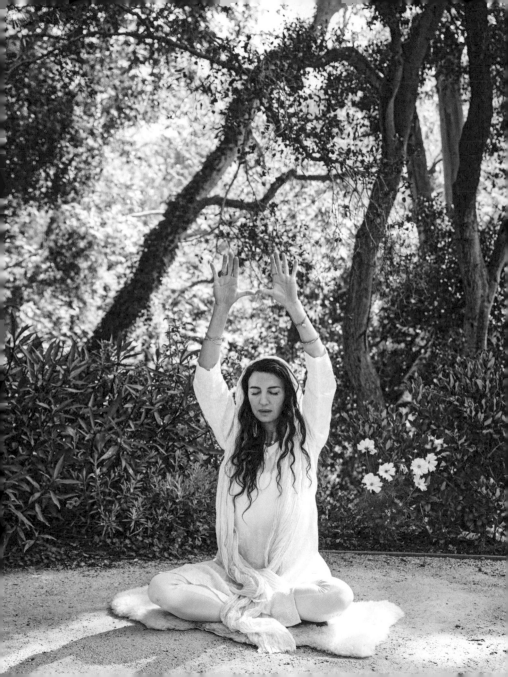

Do this for three minutes. Your arms might start to burn, but they're not going to fall off. After three minutes, bring your thumbs together so that they touch overhead, and uncurl your fingers so that they are pointing up. Tighten up your pelvic floor (almost like you're stopping the flow of urine), which will enable all of the energy you've collected to spiral up your spine toward your head.

This kriya will clean your digestive system and bring new energy and oxygen to your brain and bloodstream, all in just three minutes that will leave you with a new vitality for the rest of the day. Over time, it can change your cells.

Alternate Nostril Breathing

Alternate nostril breathing, or *nadi shodhana*, has powerful beautifying effects. *Nadi* means "energy channel" and *shodhana* means "cleaning" or "purifying." This technique keeps the mind calm and releases tension and fatigue. The alternate breathing cleanses your lungs, which oxygenates the skin, brightens the eyes, opens energy channels, and promotes better sleep. Alternate nostril breathing gets the two sides of the body to work together. The left side is the feminine nurturing, calming side and the right side is the masculine active, competitive side.

First, use your right thumb to close off your right nostril. Then inhale slowly through your left nostril. Pause for a second with your lungs full. Now close your left nostril with the ring finger of your right hand, and take your thumb off your right nostril. Exhale through your right nostril.

Begin the cycle again by inhaling through your right nostril. Pause again when your lungs are full. Use your right thumb to close off your right nostril, release your left nostril, then breathe out through your left nostril. This is one round.

Start slowly with one or two rounds and gradually increase. Never force your breath, especially if you have a stuffy nose or blocked sinuses. Sit quietly for a few moments after you have finished.

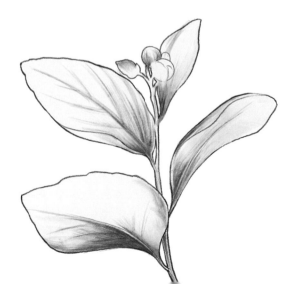

Mantras

Mantras are the sound component of Kundalini, and they are based on the concept of like attracting like. When you speak or chant a mantra, it will help bring the spirit of the mantra into your life. Mantras help rewire the brain so that the neurons fire in pathways that strengthen the body, not deplete it. In short, they help the brain get into a groove more easily, and eventually that groove becomes automatic. The mantras replace the same negative thought patterns that we repeat over and over, the ones that wear us out and create anxiety.

Kundalini mantras are thousands of years old, and they are the highest earthly vibrations that we are aware of. Most are in Gurmukhi, an ancient Indian language, but some are in English as well (see opposite). The words produce vibrations in different parts of the roof of the mouth. They activate chakras and stimulate various areas of the body and brain, and help you to listen to the sound within yourself.

MANTRAS IN ENGLISH

"I am bountiful, I am blissful,
I am beautiful."

"Happy am I, healthy am I, holy am I."

"May the longtime sun shine upon you,
all love surround you, and the pure light
within you guide your way on."

MANTRAS IN GURMUKHI

"Sat Nam."
("I am the truth.")
This is a very easy mantra and works for everyone
because its meaning is undeniable.

"Ang Sang Wahe Guru."
This mantra is not translatable, but it is the mantra
of ecstasy. Chanting it elevates the soul.

"Ong So Hung!"
("Creator, I am thou!")
This is an empowering mantra that opens the heart.

"Aad Guray Nameh."
("I bow to the primal wisdom.")
This mantra is used to invoke the protective
energy of the universe.

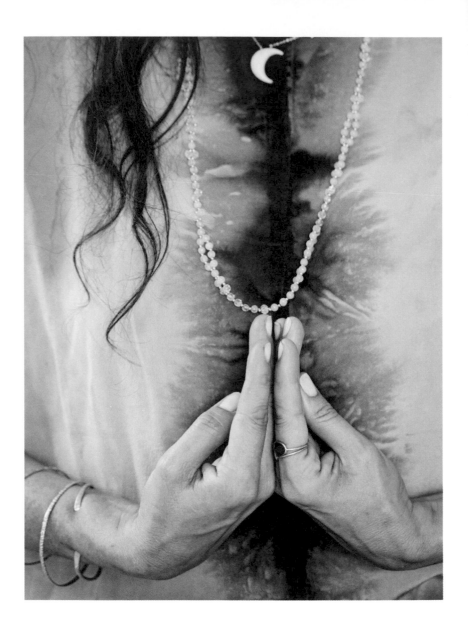

Tuning In

Tuning in is the first step before any chant or kriya. Start by putting your hands together in prayer pose, with your thumbs up against your breastbone. Bringing your hands together is like bringing together sun and moon energy, and marrying the masculine and feminine sides of yourself. Take three deep, cleansing breaths, inhaling through your nose and exhaling through your mouth.

Repeat the Adi mantra, "*Ong Namo Guru Dev Namo*," three to five times. It means "I bow to all that is the divine wisdom within myself," and it connects us to what is known as the "Golden Chain," the lineage of Kundalini masters before us. It also opens our spiritual channel so that we may receive the wisdom of the practice and connect with the source of all being.

Cat-Cow Pose

This easy yoga pose wakes up the pituitary gland, the digestion, and the spirit. The pituitary gland is about the size of a pea and is located at the base of the brain. It acts as a main control center to send messages to the other glands and is called "the seat of the mind" since it connects us to our intuition and artistry. Cat-cow is a good pose to do first thing in the morning to set the feeling for the day and connect to the source of all being. It also aids in unblocking channels so that energy can flow freely between the higher and lower chakras. According to Guru Jagat, cat-cow helps to pump cerebrospinal fluid through your spine, stimulating the production of collagen, which is what plumps your skin and keeps it firm.

TO DO CAT-COW POSE:

- Come onto the floor on your hands and knees. Make sure your hands are directly under your shoulders, about shoulder-width apart, and that your knees are directly under your hips, about hip-width apart.

- Inhale deeply into cow pose by arching your back to lift your head and chest up toward the sky and allowing your belly and rib cage to expand downward toward the ground.

- As you breathe out, round your spine to draw your head toward your tail, tucking your chin into your chest. Allow yourself to exhale completely, drawing your belly in and up toward your spine as you empty your lungs.

- Move between cow pose and cat pose, filling each movement with a long, full breath (inhaling into cow and exhaling into cat). Start off at a slow pace, then begin to move more fluidly as you feel yourself warming up. Go only as fast as you find comfortable.

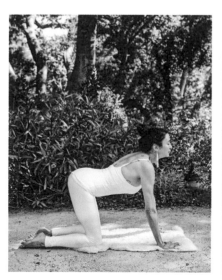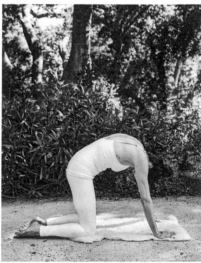

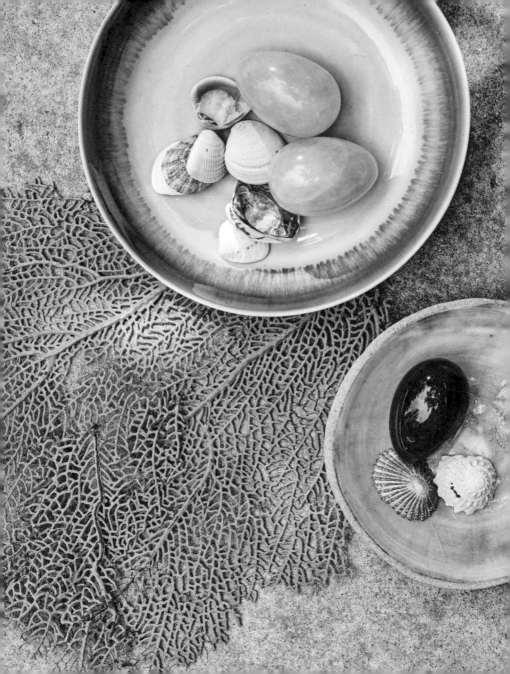

Yoni Eggs

Very rarely are women taught to honor their sexuality. Most often, we are taught to alternately fear and protect it, and it becomes a source of anxiety and feelings of inadequacy, not pleasure. But this is an exciting time because women are discovering ancient practices that can help them connect to their inner power.

Using a yoni egg is a mindfulness practice—the yoni is where many women connect with their intuition, their power, and their wisdom. It is this inner sanctum that we can access when it is not in use creating life. The word *yoni* means "sacred space" and is the symbol of the goddess, or Shakti, in Hinduism. The practice of yoni eggs was started by the empresses and concubines of ancient China. The yoni practice has so many benefits: strengthening the pelvic floor, maintaining healthy reproductive organs, and enhancing sexuality and receptiveness. It can help balance hormones, and it prevents the decline of nerves in the bladder and uterus.

More than 50 percent of women in the United States have a problem with incontinence or having orgasms. Because these subjects are not often discussed, there is some controversy surrounding the yoni egg practice, which is to be expected when dealing with an intimate topic. There is plenty of information out there, and differing views on the subject, so I feel that every woman can do her research and listen to her own intuition when deciding if the practice is for her. Sadly, you rarely hear the kind of outrage that has been directed at yoni eggs directed at other things women place in their yonis, such as dildos made with phthalates, BPA, and toxic plastics, or tampons made with pesticide-laced inorganic cotton. To me, those things are way more frightening than a beautiful yoni egg. The important issue, though, is to make sure you learn from a certified expert, like Saida Désilets or Layla Martin, and purchase *only* real gem yoni eggs (both Saida and Layla sell them through their websites; see Resources). You are placing this gem inside your sacred space, so you want to ensure that it contains all the powerful elements of the precious stones and nothing fake. You also need to make sure it is cared for and kept clean. Traditionally, yoni eggs are made from nephrite jade, which is why they're often referred to as jade eggs. I prefer jade, and many experts recommend it, but some women also use rose quartz or black obsidian.

Don't get frustrated if you don't feel anything happen right away. It takes around a month of daily use to really start perceiving the results. It is important to respect the power and sacredness of this space and practice.

CREATING A RITUAL
AROUND YOUR YONI EGG

First, cleanse and clear your egg. Boil it for
five minutes in filtered water. Dry it off and burn
some sage around it. Imagine the sage clearing
any negative feelings you might have about
your sexuality or yourself. Visualize golden
light filling the egg with positivity.

In front of your altar, or in another quiet,
private space, place the egg before you on
a beautiful scarf or piece of fabric.

Lie down on your back and place the egg
on your heart, then on your belly. Imagine
all of your intentions flowing into the egg.
Connect with it, honor it, and give thanks
for the healing it will bring you.

Follow with the exercises you have gotten
from books or an expert. Specific instructions
come with each egg, explaining exactly how to
insert it. Don't get discouraged—remember,
it's a practice. It is vital to follow all tightening
with release, since the idea of release and
expansion is at the heart of the practice.

When you're finished, clean the egg with warm
water, wrap it in silk, and store it on an altar.
It should take a sacred place in your life.

Tea Ceremony

The tea ceremony is another mindfulness practice, the purpose of which is to slow down enough that you become one mind that is fully present and in the moment. You have to be totally present as the water boils, as the leaves steep, and as you pour and drink the tea.

I practice tea ceremony with an organization called Global Tea Hut, and my teacher, Wu De, often talks about the tea ceremony as a way of connecting to nature. Many of us live in fast-paced urban environments and often fail to take notice of the natural world around us. The tea ceremony allows us to slow down enough to connect with the spirit of the earth.

Wu De taught me a simplified version of the traditional Japanese tea ceremony. Ancient Chinese and Japanese ceremonies celebrate nature by incorporating all of the elements: water, the fire and air used to boil the water, and the earth, represented by the clay cups and the tea itself. Sometimes we will also burn incense during the ceremony to represent ether. Tea is a medicine, and it brings people together. It makes it possible to sit down with a stranger, share a cup, and develop a connection without saying a word.

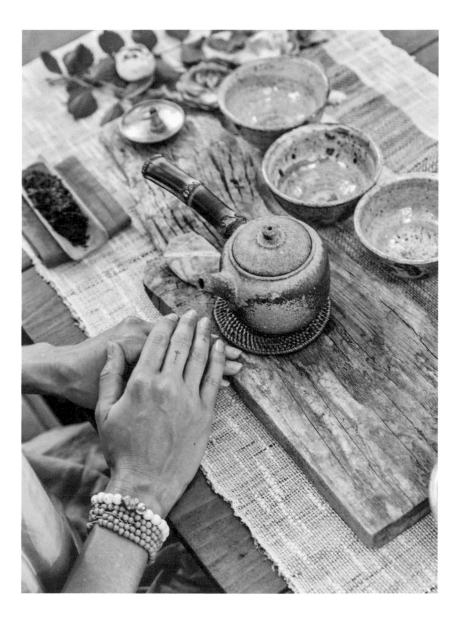

Starting your own tea practice is very simple, and you don't need much equipment. Begin with organic tea from a reliable source such as Global Tea Hut or Living Tea (see Resources) and clay cups/bowls that are nontoxic and pleasing to you.

I was introduced to the way of tea—*cha dao*—by my tea sister Tien Wu (Baelyn Elspeth), and it took me years of being the water bearer for her before I felt confident enough to serve tea. Although the practice is very simple and made for anyone to do, it also requires specific steps that come from putting in the hours to learn and absorb all of the details.

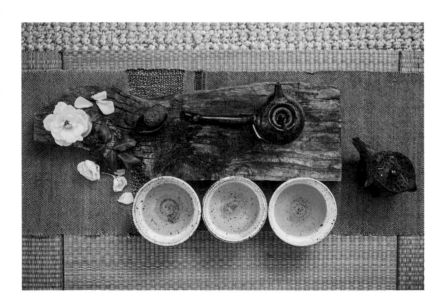

Practicing Tea Ceremony

YOU WILL NEED:

- Spring water
- A teakettle
- A nontoxic clay teapot
- Nontoxic clay teacups (Global Tea Hut sells beautiful cups and teapots that are handmade by artisans in China; see Resources)
- Organic tea
- Incense
- An offering (like a flower in a vase) that helps to decorate the space for the ceremony

TO PREPARE THE TEA:

Heat the water in a traditional teakettle until it is just about to boil, then transfer it to the teapot that you will use for the ceremony.

Put a few tea leaves in each cup/bowl, and watch them unfurl when you pour in the hot water. As with every practice, preparing tea becomes a ritual when you bring in mindfulness and intention. As the tea blossoms, really take in the history of what you are drinking. Sit outside if you can, and empty your mind of everything else by paying attention to what is around you: the sounds of nature, the feel of the warm cup in your hand, and the taste of the tea on your tongue. Sip in silence. When you are done, make an offering to tea and the earth by tossing your leaves on the ground, rather than in the trash.

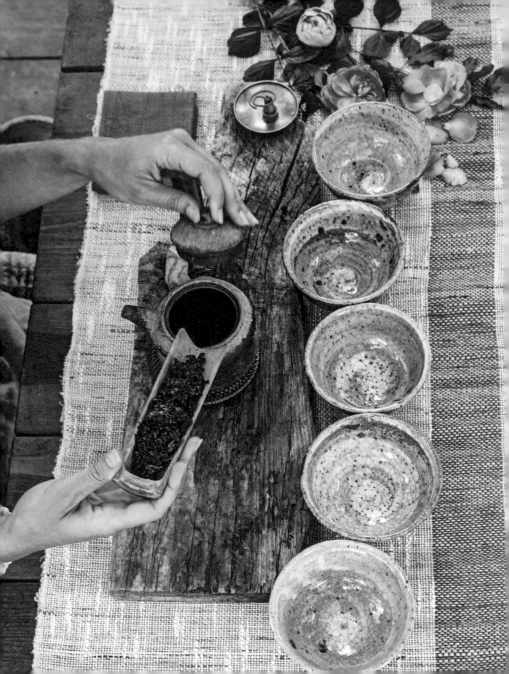

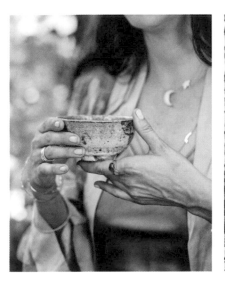
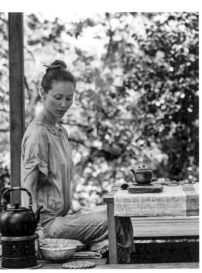

I hope that this book will serve as a bridge to a new place of spirituality and beauty—and a return to our true state of being, which is alive, healthy, blissful, vibrant, and whole.

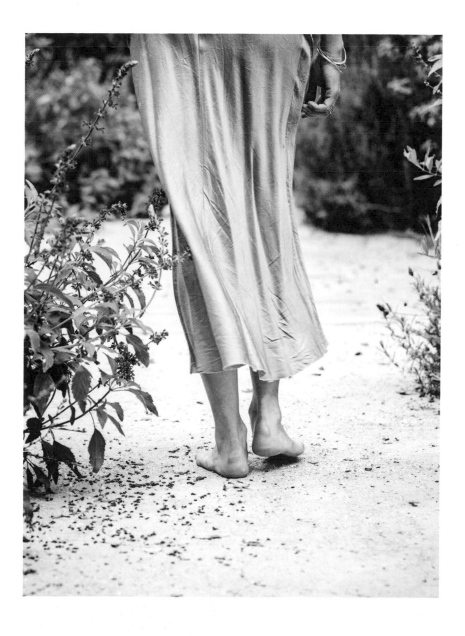

FURTHER READING

In addition to in my blog, *The Local Rose*, my
writing has appeared on the following websites.

TheChalkboardMag.com
Goop.com
MindBodyGreen.com

These are a few books I recommend.

*Awakening Shakti: The Transformative Power of the
Goddesses of Yoga*, by Sally Kempton

*Ayurvedic Beauty Care: Ageless Techniques to Invoke
Natural Beauty*, by Melanie Sachs

*Invincible Living: The Power of Yoga, the Energy of
Breath, and Other Tools for a Radiant Life*,
by Guru Jagat

Magical Herbalism: The Secret Craft of the Wise, by
Scott Cunningham

RESOURCES

Learn more about holistic living and my products on TheLocalRose.com. In addition, these are the websites I frequently visit to shop for ingredients and seek out new insights and information.

Ayurveda
BanyanBotanicals.com
Chopra.com
SuryaSpa.com

To find an Ayurvedic practitioner in your area:
AyurvedaNAMA.org

Herbs
BanyanBotanicals.com
DualSpices.com
MountainRoseHerbs.com
SusunWeed.com

Incense
Bodha.com
EarthAndElement.com

Kundalini
GoldenBridgeYoga.com
RAMAYogaInstitute.com
3HO.org

Mantras
SpiritVoyage.com
WhiteSun.com

Spices & Ingredients
BanyanBotanicals.com
DualSpices.com

Tea Ceremony
GlobalTeaHut.org
LivingTea.net

Yoni Eggs
KimAnami.com
DawnCartwright.com
Layla-Martin.com
SaidaDesilets.com

Library of Congress Cataloging-in-Publication Data

Names: Rose, Shiva, author.
Title: Whole beauty : meditation and mindfulness :
  rituals and exercises for everyday self-care / Shiva Rose.
Description: New York, NY : Artisan, a division of
  Workman Publishing Co., Inc. [2019]
Identifiers: LCCN 2018030403 | ISBN 9781579659035
  (hardcover : alk. paper)
Subjects: LCSH: Beauty, Personal. | Mind and body. | Women—
  Health and hygiene. | Self-care, Health.
Classification: LCC RA778 .R6184 2018 | DDC 613/.04244--dc23 LC
  record available at https://lccn.loc.gov/2018030403

Artisan books are available at special discounts when purchased in
bulk for premiums and sales promotions as well as for fund-raising or
educational use. Special editions or book excerpts also can be created
to specification. For details, contact the Special Sales Director at the
address below, or send an e-mail to specialmarkets@workman.com.

For speaking engagements, contact speakersbureau@workman.com.

Published by Artisan
A division of Workman Publishing Co., Inc.
225 Varick Street
New York, NY 10014-4381
artisanbooks.com

Artisan is a registered trademark of Workman Publishing Co., Inc.

This book has been adapted from *Whole Beauty* (Artisan, 2018).

Design adapted from CHD

Published simultaneously in Canada by Thomas Allen & Son, Limited

Printed in China
First printing, February 2019

10 9 8 7 6 5 4 3 2 1